Disclaimer

The information provided in this book is for educational purposes only and is not a substitute for professional medical advice. Always consult with your healthcare provider before making any changes to your diet, medication, or other health-related decisions. The content is based on general knowledge and not tailored to individual health needs. It is essential to follow your healthcare provider's recommendations and instructions. Do not disregard or delay seeking professional medical advice. The information is subject to change without notice and is provided "as is" without warranty. The authors, editors, and publishers are not responsible for any errors or omissions or for any actions taken based on the information provided.

The following information provided is intended to address potential worst-case scenarios, including situations where you may suddenly lose access to medication or treatment.

Introduction

During uncertain times, we often realize the value of things we tend to take for granted, and our health usually tops that list. Many of us and our loved ones rely on continuous medication for various health conditions. It's a scary thought to imagine a sudden disruption in the supply of medication, which got me thinking and prompted me to educate myself.

I embarked on a weight loss journey to manage my health conditions more effectively. However, I soon realized that weight loss alone might not be the ultimate solution. This realization prompted me to consider alternative forms of medication in case my prescribed medication became unavailable. To that end, I spent months researching and gathering information by consulting medical experts and reviewing medical research.

Although some of the information I gathered might be common knowledge, I appreciate that it might not be widely known. Consequently, I have compiled all the information in one place for your convenience, should you ever need to explore natural alternatives to traditional medication. I have no intention of selling you any supplements or unproven remedies. Rather, my objective is to share information about nutritious foods that are rich in vitamins and nutrients that can help fight common health conditions.

To aid in this effort, I have classified the information into various categories covering topics such as lowering blood pressure, regulating blood sugar, enhancing kidney function, maintaining cardiovascular health, safeguarding eye health, and promoting brain health. As they say, "the best defence is a good offense." Personally, I have integrated these foods and vitamins into my diet and have noticed a substantial improvement in my overall health.

In the worst-case scenario where traditional medication is not accessible, I am confident that I can cultivate or acquire and store sufficient amounts of these inexpensive ingredients and readily available vitamins to sustain my health. My aspiration is that this information will be helpful to you in the same way.

CHAPTER 1: Natural Foods That Can Help Manage Blood Pressure

1. Leafy Greens:

- Rich in nitrates which can help lower blood pressure

2. Berries:

- Rich in flavonoids that can help lower blood pressure

3. Bananas:

- Rich in potassium which can help lower blood pressure

- Studies show that increasing potassium intake can reduce blood pressure

4. Oats:

- Rich in fibre which can help lower blood pressure

- Studies show that consuming oats can reduce blood pressure

5. Garlic:

- Contains allicin which can help lower blood pressure

- Studies show that garlic can reduce blood pressure

6. Dark Chocolate:

- Rich in flavonoids that can help lower blood pressure

- Studies show that consuming dark chocolate can reduce blood pressure.

CHAPTER 2: Vitamins That Can Help Manage Blood Preesure

1. Vitamin D:

- Low levels of Vitamin D are associated with hypertension

- Studies show that increasing Vitamin D intake can lower blood pressure

2. Vitamin C:

- Acts as an antioxidant that can help reduce inflammation

- Studies show that Vitamin C can help lower blood pressure

3. Vitamin B6:

- Helps to lower homocysteine levels which can contribute to hypertension

- Studies show that Vitamin B6 can help reduce blood pressure

4. Vitamin E:

- Acts as an antioxidant that can help reduce inflammation

- Studies show that Vitamin E can help lower blood pressure

- Sources: Nuts, Seeds, Spinach

5. Potassium:

- Helps to regulate fluid balance and reduce sodium levels in the body

- Studies show that increasing potassium intake can help lower blood pressure

- Sources: Bananas, Sweet Potatoes, Avocado

6. Magnesium:

- Helps to regulate blood pressure and relax blood vessels

- Studies show that increasing magnesium intake can help lower blood pressure

- Sources: Spinach, Almonds, Cashews

7. Calcium:

- Helps to regulate blood pressure and improve blood vessel function

- Studies show that increasing calcium intake can help lower blood pressure

8. Zinc:

- Helps to improve blood vessel function and reduce inflammation

- Studies show that increasing zinc intake can help lower blood pressure

- Sources: Oysters, Beef, Chickpeas

9. Sodium:

- High levels of sodium can contribute to hypertension

- Reducing sodium intake can help lower blood pressure

- Sources: Processed Foods, Fast Foods, Salt

CHAPTER 3: Supplements That Can Help Manage Blood Pressure

1. Omega-3 Fatty Acids:

- Helps to reduce inflammation and improve blood vessel function

- Studies show that taking omega-3 supplements can help lower blood pressure

2. Coenzyme Q10 (CoQ10):

- Helps to improve blood vessel function and reduce inflammation

- Studies show that taking CoQ10 supplements can help lower blood pressure

3. L-Arginine:

- Helps to increase nitric oxide levels in the body which can improve blood vessel function

- Studies show that taking L-Arginine supplements can help lower blood pressure

4. Magnesium:

- As mentioned earlier, increasing magnesium intake can help lower blood pressure

CHAPTER 4: Lifestyle Changes That Can Help Manage Blood Pressure

1. Exercise:

- Regular exercise can help lower blood pressure

- Aim for at least 30 minutes of moderate exercise per day

- Examples: Brisk Walking, Swimming, Cycling

2. Weight Management:

- Being overweight or obese can contribute to hypertension

- Losing weight can help lower blood pressure

- Aim for a healthy body mass index (BMI)

3. Stress Management:

- Chronic stress can contribute to hypertension

- Practices like meditation, yoga, and deep breathing can help manage stress

- Aim for at least 10-15 minutes of stress-reducing activities per day

4. Quit Smoking:

- Smoking can contribute to hypertension

- Quitting smoking can help lower blood pressure

5. Limit Alcohol Intake:

- Excessive alcohol intake can contribute to hypertension

- Limit alcohol intake to 1-2 drinks per day

CHAPTER 5: Foods That Can Help Promote Eye Health

1. Leafy Greens:

- Contains lutein and zeaxanthin, which can help reduce the risk of macular degeneration and cataracts

- Sources: Spinach, Kale, Collard Greens

2. Fatty Fish:

- Contains omega-3 fatty acids, which can help reduce the risk of age-related macular degeneration

- Sources: Salmon, Tuna, Mackerel

3. Nuts and Seeds:

- Contains vitamin E, which can help reduce the risk of age-related macular degeneration

- Sources: Almonds, Sunflower Seeds, Hazelnuts

4. Citrus Fruits:

- Contains vitamin C, which can help reduce the risk of cataracts

- Sources: Oranges, Grapefruits, Lemons

5. Carrots:

- Contains beta-carotene, which can help reduce the risk of macular degeneration and cataracts

- Sources: Carrots, Sweet Potatoes, Butternut Squash

CHAPTER 6: Foods That Can Help Support Kidney Function

1. Berries:

- Contains antioxidants, which can help protect the kidneys from damage

- Sources: Blueberries, Cranberries, Strawberries

2. Fatty Fish:

- Contains omega-3 fatty acids, which can help reduce inflammation in the kidneys

- Sources: Salmon, Tuna, Mackerel

3. Garlic:

- Contains compounds that can help reduce inflammation and protect the kidneys from damage

- Sources: Fresh Garlic, Garlic Supplements

4. Whole Grains:

- High fiber intake can help reduce the risk of kidney disease

- Sources: Brown Rice, Whole Wheat Bread, Quinoa

5. Low-Fat Dairy:

- Contains calcium and vitamin D, which can help reduce the risk of kidney disease

- Sources: Low-Fat Milk, Yogurt, Cheese

CHAPTER 7: Supplements That Can Help Support Kidney Function

1. Vitamin D:

- Can help reduce the risk of kidney disease

- Sources: Supplements

2. B Vitamins:

- Can help reduce the risk of kidney disease

- Sources: Supplements

3. Probiotics:

- Can help improve gut health and reduce the risk of kidney disease

- Sources: Supplements

4. Alpha-Lipoic Acid:

- Can help reduce inflammation and protect the kidneys from damage

- Sources: Supplements

5. Cordyceps:

- Can help improve kidney function

- Sources: Supplements

CHAPTER 8: FOODS THAT CAN HELP SUPPORT LIVER FUNCTION

1. Cruciferous Vegetables:

- Contains compounds that can help detoxify the liver

- Sources: Broccoli, Cauliflower, Brussels Sprouts

2. Berries:

- Contains antioxidants, which can help protect the liver from damage

- Sources: Blueberries, Cranberries, Strawberries

3. Fatty Fish:

- Contains omega-3 fatty acids, which can help reduce inflammation in the liver

- Sources: Salmon, Tuna, Mackerel

4. Coffee:

- Contains compounds that can help reduce the risk of liver disease

5. Nuts:

- Contains compounds that can help reduce the risk of liver disease

- Sources: Walnuts, Almonds, Pistachios

CHAPTER 9: Supplements That can Help Support Liver Function

1. Milk thistle: contains silymarin which protects liver cells and promotes their regeneration.

2. Vitamin E: a powerful antioxidant that protects the liver from oxidative stress and improves liver function.

3. Vitamin C: an antioxidant that reduces inflammation in the liver and supports glutathione production.

4. B vitamins: support liver function by converting food into energy and aiding in detoxification.

5. Magnesium: reduces liver inflammation and supports glutathione production.

6. Zinc: protects liver cells from damage and aids in metabolism.

7. Selenium: important for liver function and protects against oxidative stress.

8. Betaine: found in beets and promotes liver function by reducing inflammation and promoting liver cell regeneration.

Chapter 10: Foods That Can Help Lower Blood Pressure (sources)

1. Berries:

- A study published in the Journal of the Academy of Nutrition and Dietetics found that consuming a high amount of berries was associated with a lower risk of hypertension. (1)

2. Leafy Greens:

- A study published in the Journal of Human Hypertension found that consuming leafy greens was associated with a lower risk of hypertension. (2)

3. Beets:

- A study published in the Journal of Nutrition found that drinking beet juice was associated with a significant reduction in blood pressure. (3)

4. Garlic:

- A meta-analysis of 11 randomized controlled trials found that garlic supplementation was associated with a significant reduction in both systolic and diastolic blood pressure.

5. Dark Chocolate:

- A meta-analysis of 35 randomized controlled trials found that consuming dark chocolate was associated with a significant reduction in blood pressure.

Chapter 11: More known Vitamins and Minerals That Are Known To Help Lower Blood Pressure

1. Potassium:

- A meta-analysis of 33 randomized controlled trials found that increasing potassium intake was associated with a significant reduction in blood pressure.

2. Magnesium:

- A systematic review and meta-analysis of 22 randomized controlled trials found that magnesium supplementation was associated with a significant reduction in both systolic and diastolic blood pressure. (7)

3. Vitamin D:

- A systematic review and meta-analysis of 46 randomized controlled trials found that vitamin D supplementation was associated with a modest reduction in systolic blood pressure. (8)

4. Coenzyme Q10:

- A meta-analysis of 12 randomized controlled trials found that coenzyme Q10 supplementation was associated with a significant reduction in both systolic and diastolic blood pressure. (9)

5. Omega-3 Fatty Acids:

- A systematic review and meta-analysis of 70 randomized controlled trials found that omega-3 fatty acid supplementation was associated with a significant reduction in blood pressure. (10)

<u>Chapter 12: Herbal Supplements That Can Help Lower Blood Pressure</u>

1. Hawthorn:

- A systematic review and meta-analysis of 14 randomized controlled trials found that hawthorn supplementation was associated with a significant reduction in blood pressure.

2. Garlic:

- A meta-analysis of 11 randomized controlled trials found that garlic supplementation was associated with a significant reduction in both systolic and diastolic blood pressure.

3. Hibiscus:

- A systematic review and meta-analysis of 9 randomized controlled trials found that hibiscus tea was associated with a significant reduction in both systolic and diastolic blood pressure.

4. Olive Leaf Extract:

- A systematic review and meta-analysis of 5 randomized controlled trials found that olive leaf extract supplementation was associated with a significant reduction in blood pressure.

5. Cinnamon:

- A systematic review and meta-analysis of 10 randomized controlled trials found that cinnamon supplementation was associated with a modest reduction in blood pressure.

Chapter 13: Foods That Can Help Promote Eye Health

1. Leafy greens:

- leafy greens like spinach, kale, and collard greens are rich in antioxidants that can help protect the eyes from damage caused by free radicals.

2. Fish:

- fatty fish like salmon, tuna, and sardines are high in omega-3 fatty acids, which have been shown to reduce the risk of age-related macular degeneration and dry eye syndrome.

3. Eggs:

- eggs are a good source of lutein and zeaxanthin, two antioxidants that are important for maintaining healthy vision.

4. Citrus fruits:

- citrus fruits like oranges, lemons, and grapefruits are high in vitamin C, an antioxidant that can help to protect the eyes from damage caused by free radicals.

5. Nuts:

- nuts like almonds, walnuts, and peanuts are high in vitamin E, an antioxidant that can help to protect the eyes from oxidative stress.

6. Carrots:

- carrots are rich in beta-carotene, a precursor to vitamin A, which is important for maintaining healthy vision.

7. Berries:

- berries like blueberries, strawberries, and blackberries are high in anthocyanins, which are antioxidants that can help to protect the eyes from oxidative stress and improve blood flow to the eyes.

Chapter 13: 15 simple recipes using some of the foods listed above:

1. Berry and Yogurt Smoothie:

- Blend 1 cup mixed berries with 1 cup plain yogurt and 1 banana.

2. Spinach Salad:

- Toss 2 cups spinach with 1/4 cup walnuts, 1/4 cup dried cranberries, and 2 tablespoons balsamic vinaigrette.

3. Beet and Goat Cheese Salad:

- Roast 2 beets and slice them thinly. Top with crumbled goat cheese and a drizzle of olive oil.

4. Garlic and Herb Chicken:

- Rub chicken breasts with garlic and herbs (such as thyme or rosemary) and bake at 400°F for 20-25 minutes.

5. Dark Chocolate Bark:

- Melt 1 cup dark chocolate and spread it on a baking sheet lined with parchment paper. Top with chopped nuts or dried fruit.

6. Baked Sweet Potato:

- Bake a sweet potato at 400°F for 45-50 minutes. Top with a dollop of Greek yogurt and a sprinkle of cinnamon.

7. Banana and Peanut Butter Smoothie:

- Blend 1 banana with 1 tablespoon peanut butter, 1 cup almond milk, and a handful of ice.

8. Hibiscus Tea:

- Brew hibiscus tea bags in hot water and sweeten with honey or stevia.

9. Garlic and Herb Roasted Vegetables:

- Toss chopped vegetables (such as broccoli, cauliflower, and carrots) with garlic and herbs (such as oregano or thyme) and roast at 400°F for 20-25 minutes.

10. Salmon and Quinoa Bowl:

- Cook quinoa according to package instructions and top with cooked salmon, chopped avocado, and a squeeze of lemon.

11. Blueberry Chia Seed Pudding:

- Mix 1/2 cup chia seeds with 2 cups almond milk and 1/2 cup blueberries. Let sit in the fridge for at least 2 hours.

12. Almond Butter and Banana Toast:

- Toast a slice of bread and top with almond butter and sliced banana.

13. Greek Yogurt Parfait:

- Layer Greek yogurt with mixed berries and granola.

14. Cinnamon Apple Oatmeal:

- Cook oatmeal according to package instructions and top with sliced apples and a sprinkle of cinnamon.

15. Spinach and Feta Omelette:

- Whisk together 2 eggs with a handful of spinach and crumbled feta cheese. Cook in a non-stick pan until set.

Chapter 14: Natural remedies

a few that are believed to help with the conditions mentioned.

- Hawthorn berry: Hawthorn is believed to help lower blood pressure and improve cardiovascular health. It can be consumed as a tea or taken in supplement form.

- Garlic: Garlic is believed to help lower blood pressure and improve circulation. It can be consumed raw or cooked in meals, or taken in supplement form.

- Turmeric: Turmeric is believed to have anti-inflammatory properties and may help protect against heart disease. It can be consumed in meals or taken in supplement form.

- Aloe vera: Aloe vera is believed to help improve kidney function and reduce inflammation. It can be consumed in juice form or taken in supplement form.

- Milk thistle: Milk thistle is believed to help improve liver function and protect against liver damage. It can be consumed in supplement form.

Chapter 14: Sourcing And Growing At Home

Growing your own food, herbs, and spices can be a rewarding and cost-effective way to improve your diet and incorporate beneficial nutrients into your meals. Here are some tips for growing and sourcing the foods, vitamins, and supplements mentioned above:

- Berries: Berries such as blueberries, raspberries, and strawberries are easy to grow in containers on a patio or balcony. They can also be purchased fresh or frozen at most grocery stores, and dried or powdered berry supplements can be found at health food stores or online.

- Leafy Greens: Leafy greens such as spinach and kale can be grown in a garden or in containers on a windowsill or balcony. They can also be purchased fresh at most grocery stores, and powdered greens supplements can be found at health food stores or online.

- Walnuts: Walnut trees can be grown in a garden or in a large container on a patio or balcony. Walnuts can also be purchased raw or roasted at most grocery stores, and walnut oil and supplements can be found at health food stores or online.

- Beets: Beets can be grown in a garden or in containers on a patio or balcony. They can also be purchased fresh at most grocery stores, and beet juice and supplements can be found at health food stores or online.

- Garlic: Garlic bulbs can be grown in a garden or in containers on a windowsill or balcony. Garlic can also be purchased fresh at most grocery stores: garlic supplements can be found at health food stores or online.

- Salmon: Salmon can be purchased fresh or frozen at most grocery stores, and canned salmon can be found in many stores. Fish oil supplements can also be found at health food stores or online.

- Quinoa: Quinoa can be grown in a garden or in containers on a patio or balcony. It can also be purchased dry at most grocery stores, and quinoa supplements can be found at health food stores or online.

- Chia Seeds: Chia seeds can be grown in a garden or in containers on a windowsill or balcony. They can also be purchased dry at most grocery stores, and chia seed supplements can be found at health food stores or online.

- Hibiscus: Hibiscus plants can be grown in a garden or in containers on a patio or balcony. Hibiscus tea bags can also be found in most grocery stores, and hibiscus supplements can be found at health food stores or online.

- Turmeric: Turmeric can be grown in a garden or in containers on a windowsill or balcony. It can also be purchased fresh or dried at most grocery stores, and turmeric supplements can be found at health food stores or online.

- Aloe vera: Aloe vera plants can be grown in a garden or in containers on a windowsill or balcony. Aloe vera juice can also be found in most grocery stores, and aloe vera supplements can be found at health food stores or online.

- Milk Thistle: Milk thistle can be grown in a garden or in containers on a patio or balcony. Milk thistle supplements can also be found at health food stores or online.

- When sourcing supplements, it's important to choose reputable brands and read labels carefully to ensure that the supplements are of high quality and contain the ingredients they claim to. Growing your own food can also be a fun and rewarding way to incorporate healthy foods into your diet. By growing your own produce, you can be sure of its quality and freshness, and you can save money in the process.

Chapter 15: Preserving And Storing Long Term

1. Grains: Grains such as quinoa, brown rice, and oats can be stored for long periods if kept in airtight containers in a cool, dry place. For even longer-term storage, these grains can be stored in sealed Mylar bags with oxygen absorbers.

2. Nuts: Nuts such as almonds, cashews, and walnuts can be stored in airtight containers in a cool, dark place. For even longer-term storage, nuts can be frozen or vacuum-sealed in Mylar bags.

3. Seeds: Seeds such as chia, flax, and hemp can be stored in airtight containers in a cool, dry place. For longer-term storage, seeds can be vacuum-sealed in Mylar bags.

4. Fruits and Vegetables: Fruits and vegetables can be preserved in a number of ways, including canning, dehydrating, and freezing. For canning, you will need a canning kit, which typically includes jars, lids, and a canning pot. Dehydrating can be done with a dehydrator or in the oven on low heat. For freezing, use freezer-safe bags or containers.

5. Herbs and Spices: Herbs and spices can be stored in airtight containers in a cool, dark

place. For longer-term storage, herbs and spices can be vacuum-sealed in Mylar bags.

6. Oils: Oils such as olive, coconut, and avocado can be stored in airtight containers in a cool, dark place. For even longer-term storage, oils can be stored in the freezer.

7. Vinegars: Vinegars can be stored in airtight containers in a cool, dark place. They do not require refrigeration.

The shelf life of a supplement can vary depending on the type of supplement, the storage conditions, and the packaging. Generally, most supplements have a shelf life of around 1-2 years from the date of manufacture. However, some supplements, such as probiotics, may have a shorter shelf life due to their sensitivity to moisture and heat.

The shelf life of a supplement can be extended by storing it properly in a cool, dry place away from direct sunlight and heat. Some supplements may also benefit from being stored in the refrigerator, but it is important to check the label for specific storage instructions.

Additionally, some manufacturers may add preservatives to their supplements to extend their shelf life. However, it is important to note that preservatives may not be suitable for all individuals and may cause adverse reactions in some people.

It is always best to follow the storage instructions provided by the manufacturer and to check the expiration date before taking any supplement. If the supplement has expired, it should be discarded and not consumed. When purchasing such item always look for the longest shelf life on the packaging.

Items You May need for preservation:

1. Mason jars: Mason jars are a versatile and affordable option for storing and preserving food. They can be found at most grocery stores, home goods stores or online.

2. Canning lids and bands: These are used to seal mason jars during the canning process. They can be found at the same retailers where mason jars are sold.

3. Dehydrator: A dehydrator is used to remove moisture from foods, making them less

susceptible to spoilage. They can be purchased at home goods stores or online retailers.

4. Vacuum sealer: Vacuum sealers remove air from packaging, which helps to prevent spoilage and extend the shelf life of foods. They can be found at home goods stores or online retailers.

5. Freezer bags and containers: Freezing is a simple and effective way to preserve many foods. Freezer bags and containers can be found at most grocery stores.

6. Wax paper and plastic wrap: These are useful for wrapping and storing individual portions of food. They can be found at most grocery stores.

7. Spices and herbs: Adding spices and herbs to foods can help to preserve them and add flavor. They can be found at grocery stores, health food stores, or online retailers.

8. Vinegar: Vinegar is a natural preservative that can be used to pickle vegetables or fruits. It can be found at most grocery stores.

9. Salt: Salt is another natural preservative that can be used to cure meats or preserve vegetables. It can be found at most grocery stores.

10. Sugar: Sugar can be used to make jams, jellies, and other sweet preserves. It can be found at most grocery stores.

These items can be found at various retailers, depending on where you live. Local hardware stores, home goods stores, and natural food stores are good places to start. Online retailers such as Amazon also offer a wide selection of preserving supplies.

Breathing And Meditation

Breathing techniques and meditation can have several benefits when it comes to blood pressure management. Here are some ways in which they can help:

Reducing stress and anxiety: Stress and anxiety are known to contribute to high blood pressure. Breathing techniques and meditation can help to reduce stress and promote feelings of calm and relaxation, which can help to lower blood pressure.

Improving cardiovascular function: Certain breathing techniques, such as slow, deep breathing, have been shown to improve cardiovascular function by increasing oxygen intake, reducing heart rate, and improving blood flow. This can help to reduce the workload on the heart and lower blood pressure.

Enhancing relaxation response: Meditation can help to activate the relaxation response, which is the body's natural mechanism for reducing stress and promoting relaxation. This response can help to lower blood pressure and improve overall cardiovascular health.

Reducing inflammation: Chronic inflammation is a known risk factor for high blood pressure and cardiovascular disease. Some studies have suggested that meditation can help to reduce inflammation in the body, which can have a positive effect on blood pressure.

Overall, breathing techniques and meditation can be effective tools for managing blood pressure and promoting cardiovascular health. However, it is important to consult with a healthcare professional before starting any new exercise or meditation program, especially if you have a history of high blood pressure or other medical conditions.

In An Emergency Situation

1. Call for emergency medical help: If you have access to a phone, call the emergency services in your area immediately. Even if you cannot speak, the operator can still trace your location and send help.

2. Try to stay calm and relaxed: It is important to try and stay calm, as stress and anxiety can worsen the symptoms of a stroke. Focus on your breathing and try to relax your muscles.

3. Stay in a safe position: If you feel dizzy or unsteady, sit or lie down on the floor to avoid falling and injuring yourself.

4. Do not take any medication: Do not take any medication or drink any fluids, as this can interfere with medical treatment.

5. Try to communicate: If you are able to, try to communicate with anyone who is nearby, such as a neighbour or passer-by, and ask them to call for help.

Remember, time is of the essence when it comes to stroke treatment. If you experience any of the symptoms of a stroke, such as sudden weakness or numbness in the face, arm, or leg, or difficulty speaking or understanding speech, it is important to seek medical attention as soon as possible.

Be Prepared

Being prepared highlights the importance of being well-prepared for unexpected emergencies and challenges in life. In essence, being prepared means anticipating potential challenges and taking steps to mitigate their impact in advance.

Preparedness can take many forms, depending on the situation. For example, in the case of natural disasters such as hurricanes or earthquakes, preparedness might involve creating a survival kit with essential supplies such as food, water, and medical supplies, as well as having a plan in place for evacuation or seeking shelter.

In the case of personal safety, preparedness might involve learning self-defense techniques, having a safety plan in place for situations such as home invasions or assaults, or carrying pepper spray or other protective devices.

In addition to physical preparedness, being mentally and emotionally prepared is also important. This might involve learning coping skills and stress-management techniques, developing resilience, and having a positive mind-set.

Being well-prepared can help to reduce the impact of unexpected events and increase the chances of survival. It can also reduce the likelihood of panic or poor decision-making during a crisis. By being prepared, individuals can take control of their own safety and well-being, and be better equipped to handle whatever challenges come their way.

Food preparedness is an essential aspect of overall preparedness, as access to food is critical for survival in times of emergency or crisis. Here are some key considerations for food preparedness:

1. Stock up on non-perishable food items: In an emergency situation, access to fresh food may be limited or even impossible. It is important to have a supply of non-perishable food items such as canned goods, dried fruits and nuts, and long-lasting packaged foods such as granola bars and crackers.

2. Consider dietary needs: If you have specific dietary needs or restrictions make sure to stock up on foods that meet those needs. For example, if you are vegetarian or vegan, make sure to have a supply of non-perishable plant-based proteins such as beans and lentils.

3. Store food properly: Proper storage of food can help to extend its shelf life and prevent spoilage. Keep non-perishable items in a cool, dry place away from direct sunlight. Rotate your food supply regularly to ensure that items do not expire.

4. Have cooking supplies on hand: In addition to
    food, it is important to have the necessary
    cooking supplies on hand, such as a camping
    stove or portable grill, along with fuel and
    matches.

5. Plan for water: In addition to food, access to
    clean water is essential for survival. Make sure
    to have a supply of bottled water on hand, and
    consider investing in a water filtration system
    or water purification tablets.

Overall, food preparedness is an important aspect
of overall preparedness, and taking the time to
stock up on non-perishable food items and
necessary cooking supplies can help to ensure your
survival in times of emergency or crisis.

As a compassionate and helpful person, it is
natural to want to assist others during times of
emergency or crisis. However, it is important to
exercise caution and consider your own safety and
that of your family when sharing resources in
these situations.

If you have stockpiled supplies such as food and
medication, it is important to keep this
information private. While it may be tempting to
share your preparations with friends and family, it
is wise to limit the amount of information you

divulge, particularly in the presence of strangers or those who may be less prepared.

Sharing too much information about your preparations could inadvertently make you a target for looters or others who may be looking to take advantage of those who are prepared. It is important to keep in mind that your first priority is the safety and well-being of yourself and your family.

While it is important to be prepared for emergencies, it is equally important to exercise discretion and avoid drawing attention to yourself or your resources. It may be helpful to advise friends and family to also prepare for emergencies, without disclosing the details of your own preparations.

In summary, while it is commendable to want to help others during times of emergency or crisis, it is important to exercise caution and prioritize your own safety and that of your family. Keep your preparations private and share information only with trusted individuals to ensure that you are able to weather any situation that may arise. Stay informed, stay safe.

"By failing to prepare, you are preparing to fail."

- Benjamin Franklin

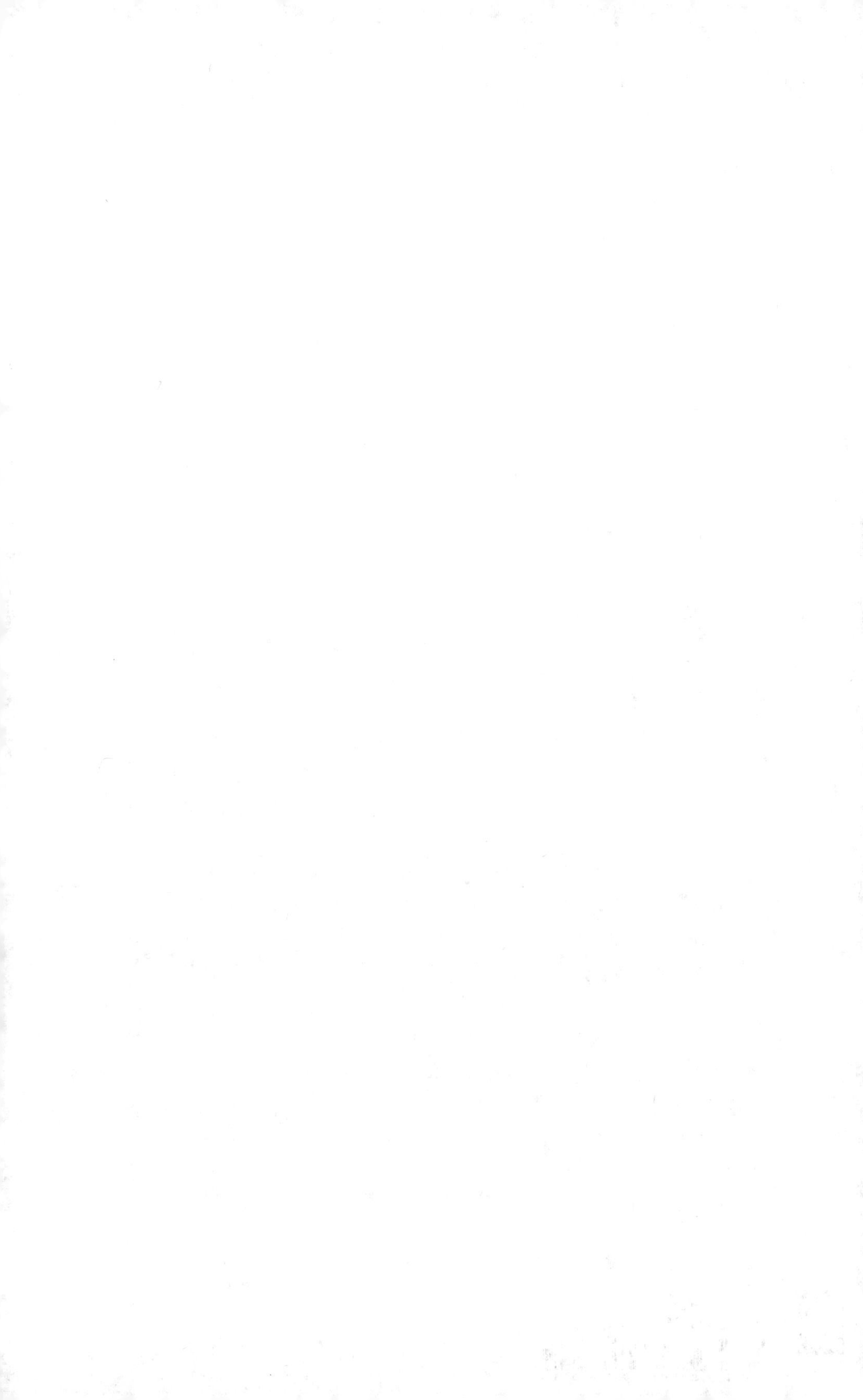